Eating the Athlete's Way

Performance-enhancing Nutritional Strategies

Table of Contents

Chapter 1. Introduction

Welcome to an exciting journey, where ordinary meals transform into powerful fuel for spectacular athletic performances! In our Special Report, "Eating the Athlete's Way: Performance-enhancing Nutritional Strategies," we delve into the seamless union of nutrition and sports, exploring how you too can harness the power of food for your athletic endeavors. Irrespective of whether you're a professional athlete, an amateur, or just someone striving for a healthier lifestyle, this report will unlock the secrets to turbocharge your performance, recovery, and overall health. It thrillingly imparts the significance of perfect nutrition timings, quality of food, and quantity for optimized performances. Wholesome, delicious, and efficient – that's the mantra we explore! Trust us; you'll want to devour every sentence as eagerly as you'll devour your next race-boosting meal after reading our special report!

Chapter 2. Unlocking the Power of Nutrition for Athletic Performance

Balancing rigorous training and adequate nutrition is the cornerstone of a successful athletic endeavor. Without proper fuel, the body cannot function at its peak, leading to decreased performance and potential injury. So how can you tap into the power of nutrition to enhance your athletic performance? Let's dive in and unlock the secrets together!

2.1. The Physiology of Sports Performance

Understanding the basic principles of sports physiology is the first step in determining the type of nutrition required. During any physical activity, the body primarily utilizes carbohydrates and fats as energy sources. How it uses these macronutrients depends largely on the intensity and duration of the exercise.

During high-intensity, short-duration activities (like sprinting), the body relies more on carbohydrates. During low-intensity, long-duration activities (like marathon running), the body also uses fat for fuel. Notably, protein plays an essential role in repairing and rebuilding muscle tissue, especially after strength and endurance training sessions.

Keeping these principles in mind, we will further highlight the importance and timing of nutrient intake to optimize sports performance.

2.2. Carbohydrates: Fast Energy Provider

Carbohydrates, or carbs, are essential for athletic performance as they provide immediate energy. Once consumed, carbs break down into glucose to fuel your muscles during exercise, with any leftover glucose stored as glycogen in the liver and muscles for later use.

Before activity: Consuming carbs 3-4 hours before training can increase glycogen stores in the body, providing more fuel for your workout. Choices like whole grains, fruits, and vegetables are excellent sources of complex carbs.

During activity: For prolonged endurance events or high-intensity training lasting more than an hour, consuming 30-60 grams of carbs per hour can maintain blood glucose levels.

After activity: Post-exercise, consume carbs within 30 minutes to replenish glycogen stores. Combining carbs with protein can enhance this effect by stimulating insulin release, which promotes glycogen synthesis.

2.3. Protein: Building and Repairing Muscle

Protein primarily serves to repair and build muscle tissues after a gruelling workout. Without sufficient protein, your muscles might struggle to recover, leading to poor subsequent performances.

After activity: After a hard workout, consuming 20-30 grams of protein can facilitate muscle recovery and promote muscle protein synthesis. High-quality proteins contain all the essential amino acids needed for this process – examples include lean meat, fish, eggs, dairy, and tofu.

During the day: Consuming protein-rich meals throughout the day can keep your body in a positive protein balance, promoting muscle growth and repair.

2.4. Fats: For Endurance Training

While fats are a less accessible energy source, they become particularly important during prolonged exercise when glycogen stores begin to deplete. High-quality fats, such as unsaturated fats, also provide essential fatty acids and fat-soluble vitamins.

During the day: To support optimal health and performance, aim for a moderate fat intake, with a focus on sources of unsaturated fats like avocados, nuts, seeds, olives, and oily fish.

2.5. Hydration: A Key to Performance

Just a 2% loss of body weight through sweat can affect performance by increasing fatigue and decreasing cognitive function. Hydrating before, during, and after exercise is thus essential to maintain optimal function and performance.

Before, during and after activity: An individual's hydration needs can vary significantly based on factors like sweat rate and exercise duration. A general rule is to consume 500-600 ml of fluid 2-3 hours before exercise, 150-200 ml every 10-20 minutes during exercise, and sufficiently after exercise to replace lost fluids.

2.6. Nutrient Timing: When You Eat Matters

Nutrient timing refers to the concept of consuming nutrients at specific times to optimize sports performance and recovery. Pre-exercise meals or snacks help to fuel your workout, post-exercise nutrition supports recovery, and meals throughout the day promote ongoing repair and adaptation.

By understanding and implementing these concepts, athletes can significantly influence their performance, recovery, and overall health, unlocking the true power of nutrition for athletic performance. The key lies not only in what you eat but when and how you consume your energy.

Just remember this: fuelling your body for performance is a marathon, not a sprint. It requires patience, experimentation, and a commitment to sustaining good eating habits over time. Bon appétit, athletes!

Chapter 3. Decoding the Athlete's Plate: Macronutrients and Micronutrients Explored

Understanding the fundamental constituents of an athlete's meal plan is the first step on the road to optimized performance. In the capacious realm of sports nutrition, two types of nutrients hold key roles: macronutrients and micronutrients. Both are needed in varying amounts, but each has a distinct and essential function in the body, and knowing how to manipulate the intake of these nutrients can drastically enhance athletic performances.

3.1. Macronutrients Explored

Macronutrients are nutrients required in large amounts in the diet. They are the powerhouse of energy and are essentially the building blocks of the body. They are divided into three categories: carbohydrates, proteins, and fats.

Carbohydrates are the primary fuel for your muscles and brain. During high-intensity exercise, the body extracts energy from carbohydrates primarily stored as glycogen in our muscles. As an athlete, it's crucial to ensure consumption of adequate complex carbohydrates, like whole grains, root vegetables, and fresh fruits to keep muscle glycogen stores filled.

Proteins, on the other hand, are vital for recovery and muscle building. Consuming adequate protein after a workout aids in repairing damaged muscles and promotes the growth of new muscle tissue. Optimal protein sources include lean meats, fish, eggs, legumes, and dairy products. As a rule of thumb, an athlete typically requires 1.2-2 grams of protein per kilogram of body weight each day, depending on the intensity and type of training performed.

Fats are also essential for athletes. They are a concentrated source of energy, providing essential fatty acids that support brain development, inflammation control, and blood clotting. Oleic and linoleic acids found in avocado, nuts, seeds, and fatty fish are all excellent sources. Be aware that while fats are needed, they should be ingested in moderation as they are high in calories and can contribute to unwanted weight gain if not balanced with expenditure.

3.2. Micronutrients Explored

Micronutrients, although required in considerably smaller amounts than macronutrients, play significant roles in body function and maintaining optimal health. They include vitamins and minerals that can't be synthesized by the body and hence, must be obtained from our diet.

Vitamins are organic compounds that aid in several body functions, including metabolism regulation, antibody production, and cell and tissue health. They are further divided into fat-soluble vitamins (vitamins A, D, E and K) and water-soluble vitamins (vitamin C and B-vitamins). Fresh fruits and vegetables, nuts, seeds, lean meats, and fish are excellent sources of vitamins.

Minerals, in contrast, are inorganic substances required for numerous body functions, from muscle contraction and nerve function to bone health and fluid balance. Calcium, Iron, potassium, and magnesium are some important minerals for athletes. Calcium is necessary for bone health and muscle function, iron supports oxygen transportation, potassium aids in muscle contractions and supports heart health, while Magnesium is crucial for energy production and supporting nerve and muscle function.

3.3. The Right Mix: Striking the Balance

One of the challenges most athletes grapple with is striking the right balance between macronutrients and micronutrients. It's not just about consuming these nutrients; it's also about when and how to consume them to optimize athletic performance. Timing and balance are critical factors. For instance, consuming carbohydrates more heavily around workouts can enhance energy levels, while also ensuring replenishment of lost glycogen stores. Similarly, consuming protein post-workout aids in muscle recovery and growth.

The suitable ratio of macronutrients is another factor to consider. The ideal plate of an athlete may comprise roughly 45–65% of calories from carbohydrates, 10–30% from protein, and 20–35% from fat, according to the Dietary Guidelines for Americans. These ratios may vary based on individual needs, the type of sport or training, and the athlete's goals.

Micronutrient needs may also vary based on the athlete's gender, body size, age, and training intensity. For instance, high-intensity and long-duration exercises may heighten the need for B-vitamins and antioxidants to assist with energy metabolism and repair from oxidative stress.

In conclusion, achieving the right balance of macronutrients and micronutrients is essential for athletes for optimal performance. Paying attention to the quality of food, the timing of consumption, and ideal proportions can drastically improve training outcomes, enhance recovery, and bolster overall health.

Chapter 4. Timing is Everything: The Science of Nutrient Timing

Nutrient timing is the systematic planning of food and fluid intake around the various events in an athlete's training schedule. It's a strategy that can help you get the most out of every aspect of your training and performance. Nutrition plays an integral role in optimizing performance and recovery from these sessions. The key is understanding when and what to eat to maximize these benefits.

4.1. A Basic Overview of Nutrient Timing

Athletes are constantly in a cycle of training and recovery. Training breaks down tissues, making small tears and depleting glyogen stores. While this might sound damaging, it's part of the process that eventually leads to better fitness, strength, and performance. The body responds to these training-induced stressors by rebuilding and reshaping tissues to be more resilient to the same stress in the future.

Nutrient timing focuses on when to eat, relative to exercise, to boost these restorative processes. It involves everything from when to eat before, during, and after exercise, through to the timing of meals throughout the day and even week. Simply put, nutrient timing is eating specific nutrients, such as carbohydrates and protein, in and around your workouts.

This strategy begins with a well-balanced diet which provides the necessary fuel for your training. Then, by timing your nutrients, you optimize this fuel to enhance your performance. Eating before a workout ensures your muscles have enough fuel, while consuming the right nutrients after a workout supports recovery.

4.2. Pre-Workout Nutrition

The primary goal of your pre-workout meal is to give your body the fuel it needs to maximize performance and delay the onset of fatigue. That breakout session, sprint, or workout depends on the quality of your pre-workout meal.

The timing of this meal depends on the type of fuel your body needs. Generally, a meal 3-4 hours before workout provides ample time for digestion and absorption. It should contain complex carbohydrates for sustained energy, lean protein to prepare for post-workout recovery, and healthy fats.

A small, easily digestible snack around 30-60 minutes before workout can top off your body's energy reserves. But keep in mind, too much fat or fiber, or a too-large portion may upset your stomach during the workout.

4.3. Intra-Workout Nutrition

For the endurance athlete, nutrition during exercise plays a significant role. Once your workout stretches beyond the 60-minute mark, you need to refuel. Fluids, electrolytes, and simple carbs become an athlete's sustenance in these cases.

Hydration is key. Sweat loss can lead to dehydration, which can resultantly impair performance. Electrolyte-filled sports drinks can replenish lost fluids and important minerals like sodium and potassium.

Carbohydrates are also important during prolonged exercise. The body can rapidly use these carbs to sustain energy levels, delay fatigue, and enhance performance. Ideally, 30-60g of simple carbs per hour are recommended in endurance events.

4.4. Post-Workout Nutrition

Post-workout nutrition is vital for recovery after strenuous workouts. The body's glycogen stores are depleted, muscle tissues have been broken down, and dehydration may have occurred.

Within the first 30 minutes after your workout – often called the "golden hour" – your muscles are primed for recovery. A blend of protein and carbohydrates makes the optimal post-exercise meal or snack.

Carbohydrates refill your glycogen stores for future exercise sessions. Proteins, on the other hand, provide the raw materials for muscle tissue repair and growth. Aim for a post-workout snack or meal that provides 3:1 to 4:1 ratio of carbohydrates to protein.

4.5. The Importance of Consistency

One-off nutrient-timed meals will not magically transform your performance. It's the consistent application of these strategies that yields benefits. Creating a sustainable, adaptable eating pattern that works with your training schedule is key.

Remember, everyone responds differently to foods and timings. What works best for one athlete may not work for another. The art of nutrient timing is personal; it requires experimentation, refining, and commitment. But, with persistence, this science-backed approach can greatly enhance your athletic performance and recovery.

4.6. Take-Away Points

- Nutrient timing involves eating the right foods at the right times to enhance performance and recovery.

- Proper pre-workout nutrition can maximize performance and delay the onset of fatigue.

- Adequate nutrition during prolonged workouts can help sustain energy levels, delay fatigue, and enhance performance.

- Consuming a blend of protein and carbohydrates shortly after a workout can support recovery.

- Consistency and personalization are key elements to making nutrient timing work for you.

Through understanding nutrient timing, you're not just fueling for a single workout or race. Instead, you're establishing eating patterns that sustain ongoing training, optimizing workouts today, tomorrow, and beyond. By fueling smarter, you set yourself up for better health and performance long term. After all, every good performance is simply the next workout, properly fueled and well-recovered, from the one before. It's time to let your nutrition work for you, rather than you always working for your nutrition!

Chapter 5. Fuel to Fly: Tailoring Nutrition for Endurance Athletes

In the realm of endurance sports, nutrition plays a critical role. It is not a mere supplement to an athlete's regime; rather, it forms the very foundation upon which all training, performance, and recuperation rest. A thoughtfully crafted nutritional plan indeed has the potential to make or break an athlete's performance. In this chapter, we'll understand just how to craft an effective nutrition strategy to meet the unique demands of endurance sports.

5.1. Understanding Endurance Sports

Endurance sports – be it marathon, cycling, or triathlon – demand prolonged periods of high-intensity effort from athletes. With regular workouts lasting anywhere between an hour to several hours, endurance athletes routinely push their bodies to the limit. Such grueling training and performance schedules test not just the athletes' physical prowess, but their nutritional strategy as well.

5.2. Building Blocks of an Endurance Athlete's Diet

The primary job of your diet is to provide fuel, and the main source of fuel for endurance events is carbohydrates. Stored as glycogen in the muscles and liver, carbohydrates, when converted into glucose, provide the energy you need to keep performing.

However, protein and fats, albeit in smaller amounts, also play significant roles. Protein aids in recovering muscle tissue, post-workout healing, and developing new tissues. Fats, on the other hand, can provide a substantial energy store for longer, less intense endurance events.

More accurately understanding these three pillars' intake, distribution, and timing can significantly enhance an athlete's performance and recovery.

5.3. The Right Time: Nutrient Timing

Endurance athletics demands a keen focus on "when" to eat, beyond the "what" and "how much" elements of dietary planning. Understanding optimal nutrient timing allows athletes to fuel their bodies effectively for workouts and speed up recovery post-exercise.

Before the workout, it's crucial to prioritize easily digestible carbohydrates to top off glycogen stores. During the exercise, refueling is necessary in workouts or races that go beyond one hour to replenish the energy. Post-workout nutrition targets efficient recovery, with an emphasis on carbohydrates for glycogen synthesis and protein for muscle repair.

5.4. Nutrient Distribution: Striking the Balance

Striking the correct balance of macronutrients (carbohydrates, fats, and proteins) is critical for endurance athletes. While this balance may vary based on training needs and the athlete's body composition, generally, it falls into the following distribution:

- Carbohydrates: 60-70%

- Proteins: 15-20%

- Fats: 20-25%

This distribution ensures that the body remains adequately fueled for performance and repair while minimizing any unnecessary fat gain.

5.5. Quality of Food: Choosing Your Fuel Wisely

Just as a high-performance car requires premium fuel, an athlete's body needs high-quality nutrients. Endurance athletes should aim for whole, unprocessed food with high nutrient density. Incorporating a variety of fruits, vegetables, legumes, lean meats, and whole grains can ensure the body receives a broad spectrum of necessary vitamins and minerals.

5.6. Staying Hydrated: The Essential Role of Fluids

In addition to the macronutrients, staying adequately hydrated before, during, and after an event is paramount for endurance sports. Dehydration can lead to decreased cognitive and motor function, increased heart rate, and ineffective thermoregulation – all impairing athletic performance.

5.7. Fine-tuning Your Diet with Micronutrients

While the focus so far has remained on macronutrients, we should not downplay the importance of micronutrients. These essential vitamins and minerals are indispensable for multiple physiological functions, including energy production and muscle contraction. An endurance athlete must regularly take stocks for necessary micronutrients like Iron, Calcium, Vitamin D, and B-vitamins in their diets to avoid deficiency.

5.8. Periodization in Nutrition: A Dynamic Approach to Food

Consider adopting nutritional periodization, an approach where you adjust your dietary approach based on varying demands across your training cycle. It ensures that your diet syncs with your workout demands, from lighter training periods to intense workout weeks, or even the final countdown to the race day.

5.9. Dodging Dietary Disasters: Common Pitfalls to Avoid

Abstaining from over- or under-eating, avoiding new foods or nutritional strategies close to race day, recognizing symptoms of potential eating disorders, and not relying solely on supplements can help athletes veer clear of common dietary pitfalls.

5.10. Individualization: The Key to Success

Every athlete has unique nutritional needs based on their body composition, lifestyle, training schedule, and personal preferences. Individualizing the nutrition strategy by paying attention to these nuances increases not only the athlete's comfort but can also result in notable performance gains.

Harnessing nutritional knowledge for endurance sports can provide an edge that allows athletes to train harder, recover faster, and perform better. In fueling wisely lies the power to endure and excel in your sport of choice!

Chapter 6. Strength on a Plate: Nutrition for Power and Strength Athletes

Strength athletes require optimal nourishment to perform at their best and recover faster. This chapter delves into the personalized nutritional needs of strength athletes, focusing on the macronutrients and micronutrients vital to maximize their power output and accelerate recovery.

6.1. Macronutrient Needs

Nutritional needs of strength athletes primarily revolve around three macronutrients: carbohydrates, proteins, and fats. The right balance and timing of these nutrients are crucial for strength and power development.

Carbohydrates provide the energy necessary for high-intensity workouts. However, unlike endurance athletes who rely heavily on carbs, strength athletes need a balanced mix – incorporating carbs, proteins, and fats.

The International Society of Sports Nutrition recommends a carbohydrate intake of 4-7 g/kg body weight per day for strength training athletes. This intake should be timed around their workout – notably, pre-workout and post-workout meals – to ensure optimal energy delivery and glycogen replenishment.

Proteins play a vital role in muscle repair and growth, and are important for strength athletes who undergo strenuous muscle-damaging workouts. The daily protein requirement for these athletes ranges between 1.6-2.2 g/kg body weight, spread evenly over 4-6 meals to maximize muscle protein synthesis.

Fats should not be overlooked, as they are a concentrated source of energy. A moderate fat intake – around 20-35% of total daily caloric intake – is recommended. It contains essential fatty acids and aids in the absorption of fat-soluble vitamins, promoting overall health.

6.2. Micronutrient Considerations

Micronutrients such as vitamins, minerals, and trace elements play a crucial role in numerous bodily functions, including energy production, bone health, and immune function.

Strength athletes, due to intense workouts, may have higher needs for certain vitamins and minerals. Iron, calcium, vitamin D, B-vitamins, and antioxidants should be prioritized. Iron supports oxygen transport while calcium and vitamin D promote bone health. B-vitamins aid in energy production, and antioxidants help reduce exercise-induced oxidative stress.

It's always best to meet micronutrient needs through food sources first. But in certain cases, supplementation may be necessary under professional guidance.

6.3. Hydration Strategies

For strength athletes, proper hydration is vital. Water regulates body temperature, lubricates joints, and aids in nutrient transport. It's recommended to drink enough fluids to balance any fluid lost during workouts.

In high-intensity or long duration training, athletes may lose electrolytes through sweat, which need to be replaced. A simple hydration strategy could be 500-600 ml of water 2-3 hours before exercise, 150-250 ml every 15-20 minutes during exercise, and adequate intake post-exercise to balance fluid loss.

6.4. Optimizing Meal Timing

Meal timing is a tool that can be used to maximize performance and recovery. Pre-workout meals, taken 2-3 hours before exercising, should provide sufficient carbohydrates to fuel the workout and high-quality proteins to reduce muscle protein breakdown.

Immediately post-workout, consuming a combination of simple carbohydrates and proteins can maximally stimulate muscle protein synthesis and replenish glycogen stores. A ratio of 3:1 carbs to protein can be effective.

Later, in the recovery period, balanced meals and snacks including all macronutrients should be consumed to support continued recovery and adaptation.

6.5. Supplement Considerations

Certain dietary supplements might be helpful for strength athletes. Creatine, for example, is one of the most researched supplements and has been proven to enhance strength and power development. Beta-alanine could delay muscle fatigue, and caffeine may improve workout intensity.

Before adding any supplements, it's important to consult with a healthcare provider or a skilled nutritionist, to avoid potential adverse effects or interactions.

In the pursuit of strength and power, remember that nutrition is a powerful tool. When wielded correctly, it can propel you towards your athletic goals while supporting health and recovery. Balance is key – in macronutrients, micronutrients, hydration, meal timing, and supplementation. You're not just what you eat; you're also when and how you eat! Harness the power of 'Strength on a Plate' and fuel your journey to becoming a strength athlete!

Chapter 7. The Refresh Button: Nutrition for Recovery

Performing at your peak doesn't end the moment you cross the finish line or blow the final whistle. The choices you make post-exercise can have just as significant an impact on your future performance as your in-game strategy or training regimen. As you'll soon discover, recovery nutrition is a key player in this equation, and understanding its principles can be the difference between persistently outdoing yourself and experiencing progress plateaus.

7.1. The science behind recovery

The concept of recovery nutrition is rooted in physiology. During exercise, muscles undergo stress, leading to the breakdown of glycogen stores and muscle protein. Recovery nutrition aims to replenish these stores and repair the tissue, enabling athletes to return to their optimal performance level sooner.

A balanced recovery strategy hinges on three key elements: replenishing glycogen stores with carbohydrates, repairing muscle tissue with protein, and rehydration.

1. Carbohydrates: High-intensity and long-duration exercises, such as marathons or triathlon events, drain the glycogen stores in muscles. Consuming carbohydrates after exercise restores these levels. Without sufficient replenishment, your muscles may feel fatigued, and your next session's performance could potentially take a hit.

2. Protein: Exercise breaks down muscle protein structures, necessitating repair and remodeling post-exercise. Consuming

sufficient protein after a workout provides the necessary amino acids for these processes.

3. Hydration: Sweating, a normal physiological response to exercise, can result in substantial fluid and electrolyte loss. Neglecting fluid balance can lead to dehydration, which significantly impairs both physical and cognitive performance.

7.2. The recovery window: Timing is everything

The timing of recovery nutrition can greatly influence its effectiveness. Exercise increases insulin sensitivity and blood flow to muscles, creating a so-called 'window of opportunity.' During this period, generally 30 to 60 minutes post-workout, the muscles are especially receptive to nutrients—primarily carbohydrates and proteins—that support recovery.

This doesn't mean that if you miss this window, all recovery benefits will be lost. The body continues healing and repairing itself long after a workout, but for speedy recovery, this soon-after-exercise dietary approach can be a game-changer.

7.3. Recovery fuel: What to eat

To kickstart the recovery process, focus on consuming a balance of carbohydrates and protein within two hours of exercise. Here are some optimized nutrients and their sources:

1. Carbohydrates: Opt for nutrient-dense, whole-food carbohydrate sources, such as whole grains, fruits, and starchy vegetables. Examples include rice, pasta, bread, bananas, apples, and potatoes.

2. Protein: Animal proteins, like eggs, meat, and dairy, contain all essential amino acids our bodies need but can't produce on their

own. Plant-based protein sources, while generally not as complete, can be combined to provide a full amino acid profile. Think beans and rice or hummus and whole grain bread.

3. Hydration: Drink water throughout the day, but especially before, during, and after exercise to maintain hydration. Beverage choices such as milk provide not only hydration but also key nutrients like protein and carbohydrates.

7.4. Examining practical recovery meals/snacks

Dietary preferences, intolerances, and habits can all influence what recovery foods will look like. The most important factor is that the meal or snack contains an appropriate balance of the key nutrients. Here are few examples:

- Chocolate milk: A glass provides fluid for hydration, carbohydrates for glycogen replenishment, and protein for muscle repair.

- Eggs on toast: This offers a good balance of carbohydrates through the bread and protein from the eggs.

- Yogurt with fruit and granola: Here, yogurt supplies protein, fruit provides vitamins and fiber, and granola contributes carbohydrates.

7.5. Nutrient supplementation

Supplements can be a helpful tool for athletes struggling to consume sufficient nutrients through food alone or those with limited time or specific dietary restrictions. Whey protein powders, BCAA supplements, and carbohydrate powders can all be valuable assets.

However, always remember that while supplements can enhance

your recovery strategy, they should not replace a balanced diet of whole foods.

7.6. Trial and adjustment

What works for one athlete may or may not work for another. Factors such as age, sex, training intensity, and dietary preferences all influence an individual's recovery nutrition needs. Therefore, there should be an emphasis on trial and adjustment. Experiment with different recovery foods and timing strategies to identify what works best for you. Monitor your recovery progress, how you feel, and any changes in your performance to determine your most effective nutritional strategy.

In conclusion, think of recovery nutrition as an extension of your training—a critical factor that contributes significantly to your next game's performance, your overall performance in the season, and your long-term athletic career. Optimize your nutrition, optimize your recovery, and watch as your performance reaches new heights.

Chapter 8. Hydration Station: Fluids and Athletic Performance

It's as clear as mountain spring water - hydration plays a crucial role in all human mechanisms, particularly for athletes, be they professionals or weekend warriors. Too much or too little water can negatively affect performance and health. This chapter will quench your thirst for knowledge on hydration facts, the role of different fluids, and strategies to stay optimally hydrated for your best athletic performance.

8.1. Importance of Hydration

Water constitutes about 60% of the human body. It is fundamental for all physiological processes, including digestion, absorption, transportation, dissipation of heat, and excretion of waste. For an athlete, hydration status can significantly impact physical and mental performance.

As an athlete loses water via perspiration and respiration during exercise, even a small percentage of dehydration (a 2% decrease in body water) can compromise athletic performance. These effects can be seen through reduced endurance, increased fatigue, decreased coordination, and a decline in mental sharpness. Moreover, during dehydration, body temperature and heart rate may rise, putting pressure on your body and potentially posing a risk to your health.

8.2. Types of Fluids and Their Roles

Staying hydrated isn't just about drinking water. Different fluids offer a variety of benefits essential to athletic performance.

Water: This is the primary fluid for staying hydrated. It helps maintain blood volume, keeps the body cool, and allows muscles, cardiovascular system, and brain to function correctly. However, water alone is not always sufficient, especially during intense or prolonged workouts.

Sports Drinks: Containing balanced proportions of electrolytes and carbohydrates, sports drinks are useful during prolonged, intense exercise sessions. The carbohydrates provide fuel, while electrolytes help replace what's lost in sweat and maintain fluid balance.

Fruit Juices: Packed with vitamins and minerals, fruit juices can contribute to an athlete's intake of hydration, as well as crucial nutrients for performance and recovery. However, due to their high sugar content, they should be consumed in moderation.

Herbal Teas: These can aid hydration and provide additional benefits like antioxidants and anti-inflammatory properties. Nevertheless, caffeinated teas should be consumed carefully due to their diuretic effect.

Milk: Research suggests that milk (especially chocolate milk) could be an excellent post-workout hydration source. It contains carbohydrates, proteins, and fats necessary for muscle recovery, and it hydrates more effectively than some commercially available sports drinks.

8.3. Hydration Strategies

Knowing when and how much liquid to drink can be as important as the type of fluid consumed.

Before Exercise: Consume approximately 500 ml of liquid, 2-3 hours before the workout start. This gives the kidneys adequate time to expel any excess fluid and reach a state of balanced hydration before starting exercise.

During Exercise: The general guideline is to consume about 150-200 ml of fluids every 15-20 minutes during the workout, but this varies based on factors like exercise intensity, duration, and individual sweat rate.

After Exercise: For every kilogram lost during exercise, aim to replenish it with 1.25 - 1.5 litres of fluid over the next 2-6 hours to account for the continual sweat and urine losses post-exercise.

8.4. Tips to Maintain Hydration

Monitor Your Weight: A routine weigh-in before and after workout sessions can help monitor your fluid loss. A noticeable difference in weight would suggest a significant fluid loss.

Consume Foods High in Water: Many fruits and vegetables, such as watermelon, cucumber, oranges, and strawberries, have high water contents that can contribute to your overall fluid intake.

Avoid Dehydration Triggers: Limit caffeinated beverages and alcohol, especially around your workout times. They can have a diuretic effect, promoting fluid loss.

Keep Fluids Accessible: Always keep a water bottle handy in your gym bag, at your desk, or wherever you spend significant time.

8.5. From Hydration Theory to Practice

Hydration needs are highly individual and depend on several factors such as body composition, environment, level and intensity of activity, and diet. Adopting a personalized hydration protocol, developed in consultation with a nutritionist or a sports dietitian, can help you optimize hydration for your best athletic performance. Above all, listening to your body's signals for thirst and monitoring your urine color for hydration status are the simplest and most effective real-time hydration metrics.

In conclusion, hydration is neither an art nor a science; instead, it is a delicate balance. Understanding the importance of fluid balance, the distinct roles of various fluids, and employing effective hydration strategies can fuel your body for optimal athletic performance. The dividends of being well-hydrated extend beyond your workouts: improved overall health, enhanced cognition, and a solid foundation for peak performance in all areas of life. No matter what your athletic goal, staying hydrated is the starting line in the race to success. Keep pouring, keep performing!

Chapter 9. Mastering Meal Planning: Practical Tips for Athletes

Eating optimally for sports performance is a fine balance between intake and expenditure, where quality, quantity, and timing of meals constitute a triad for success. Let's delve into the intricate details that need to be factored into your nutrition strategy, paving the way towards a practical meal plan for athlete's performance and success.

9.1. Building Your Plate

When it comes to the nutritional world, one size does not fit all. However, understanding the general layout of a healthy, balanced plate can swiftly set you on the course towards good nutrition.

Your plate should be divided into four key components:

1. 1/2 of it filled with colorful fruits and vegetables

2. 1/4 filled with whole grains

3. 1/4 filled with lean protein

4. A side serving of healthy fats

This blueprint is adjustable depending on your training regimen and overall goals–you may need more proteins during strength or resistance training days or extra carbohydrates for endurance events.

9.2. Understanding Macronutrients

The body needs macronutrients–carbohydrates, proteins, and

fats–for energy, growth, immunity and maintaining overall health. The primary macronutrient sources for an athlete should be:

1. Carbohydrates: Whole grains, fruits, vegetables; primary source of energy.

2. Proteins: Lean meats, fish, eggs, legumes, whole grains; essential for muscle repair and mass development.

3. Fats: Nuts, seeds, avocados, olives; aids in absorption of fat-soluble vitamins and provide essential fatty acids.

Remember, all meals and snacks should include a balance of macronutrients. Tailor the ratios to your activity type and levels.

9.3. Individual Energy Requirements

Individual daily energy expenditure can be remarkably variable among athletes. Factors that affect energy expenditure include your sport type, intensity, duration of workouts, body weight, and muscle mass.

To calculate your daily energy needs, you can use tools such as Harris-Benedict Equation that takes into account the Basal Metabolic Rate (BMR) and physical activity level. This estimation should be used as a starting point to develop your meal plan.

9.4. Meal Timing

Your body requires a consistent fuel supply across the day and not just during workouts. It is recommended:

1. Consuming a meal 2–4 hours before a workout, focusing on carbs and protein.

2. Eating a small snack an hour before the workout if not consumed

a meal.

3. Refueling within 30–60 minutes after intense workout with high quality protein and carbohydrate.

9.5. Hydration

Drinking fluids is crucial for maintaining physical performance. Adequate intake depends largely on activity levels and weather conditions. A general guide is 30–35 milliliters of fluid per kilogram of body weight per day. Remember to replace the fluids lost during exercise by drinking 450–675 milliliters of water per half kilogram of body weight lost.

9.6. Supplements

Supplements should be taken cautiously, and only when required. Before absolutely necessary, focus should be on achieving balanced and sufficient nutrient intake through food.

9.7. Sample Meal Plan

Here's an example of an everyday meal plan:

Breakfast: Overnight oats with chia seeds, berries, and a hard-boiled egg Snack: Greek yogurt with almonds and banana Lunch: Grilled chicken salad with dark leafy greens, cherry tomatoes, and avocado Pre-Workout: Whole wheat toast with natural peanut butter and sliced banana Post-Workout: Protein shake with a side of apple slices and almond butter Dinner: Salmon with quinoa and roasted veggies Snack: Cottage cheese with cinnamon and fresh peaches

This meal plan provides sufficient nutrients for a moderate to high intensity exercise regimen. Always adjust according to your energy needs.

9.8. Conclusion

A strategic meal plan adapted to an athlete's unique needs can be the game changer in athletic performance. Prioritize whole foods, balance macronutrients, hydrate effectively and time meals efficiently to fuel your success.

Remember, nutrition is a journey. Setting up your meal plan and adjusting it as you progress in your athletic career, listen to your body, seek guidance from a registered dietitian, and most find the most sustainable plan that aids you in achieving your peak performance.

Chapter 10. Supplementing the Athlete's Way: What Works and What Doesn't

Athletes have long sought out different ways to gain a competitive edge by enhancing physical endurance, strength, and recovery speed. One such approach includes the use of various inclusions into your dietary habits which we call supplements. It's important to note that these aren't the quick-fix solutions they're often marketed as, but rather an adjunct to an existing sound nutritional plan. The common consensus among researchers is that supplements are most effective when your regular diet is optimized to begin with.

10.1. Supplementing the Athlete's Diet: Who, Why, and When

Supplements cater to a varied audience, from high-performing professional athletes who strive to push their limits, to everyday people juggling exercise with work-life balance. While their usage is potential across a broad spectrum of activities, they're especially valued by athletes who engage in high-intensity training or endurance-based activities. Your body has a finite capacity for work, and this limit can be nudged a little further with the help of supplements.

There's no "one-size-fits-all" answer to when and why supplements should be used. It comes down to the individual's dietary needs and athletic goals. Most supplements offer a 'buffer' for when your diet isn't providing enough nutrients or to help augment performance during specific periods of training or competition.

10.2. The Good Stuff: Proven and Effective Supplements

Let's get down to brass tacks. What are some credible, science-backed supplements that can help an athlete push their boundaries?

10.2.1. Protein Supplements

Protein is the construction material for your muscles. It repairs and rebuilds muscle tissue after strenuous workouts, fostering muscle growth and recovery. Athletes often struggle to meet their recommended protein requirements through diet alone, making protein supplements like whey, casein, and plant-based proteins a worthwhile consideration.

10.2.2. Creatine

One of the most researched and proven supplements, creatine enhances muscle strength and explosive power, making it beneficial for strength and power athletes. It's a natural substance that converts into creatine phosphate in the body, aiding in the formation of ATP, our body's primary energy carrier.

10.2.3. Beta-Alanine

This is an amino acid that boosts muscular endurance, enhancing performance in high-intensity exercises lasting one to several minutes. It works by accumulating in the muscles and reducing the buildup of lactic acid during intense workouts.

10.2.4. BCAAs

Branched-Chain Amino Acids (BCAAs) are essentially three essential amino acids - leucine, isoleucine, and valine. They are directly absorbed by the muscles and can reduce muscle soreness, reduce exercise fatigue, and stimulate muscle protein synthesis.

10.3. Treading with Caution: Supplements with Mixed or Insufficient Evidence

While numerous supplements show promise in enhancing athletic performance, the jury's still out on their definitive benefits. Using these supplements requires a certain degree of caution.

10.3.1. HMB

Beta-hydroxy-beta-methylbutyrate (HMB) is a product of the amino acid leucine. Early studies suggested it might help increase strength and body composition, but later research has led to mixed results.

10.3.2. Glutamine

Athletes often use glutamine for its alleged effect on muscle recovery. While there's some evidence supporting its benefits for injury or surgery recovery, its utility in healthy athletes remains unclear.

10.3.3. Deer Antler Velvet

Marketed primarily for its IGF-1 content - a growth hormone - the claims surrounding Deer Antler Velvet for strength or endurance enhancement remain unsubstantiated by large-scale, repeated studies.

10.4. Supplements to Avoid: Potentially Harmful or Ineffective

The supplement world, fueled by aggressive marketing, is marred with products that offer little to no benefits or, worse, are potentially harmful.

10.4.1. "Boosters"

Whether they're marketed as testosterone, growth hormone, or fat 'burners,' they're commonly ineffective and can potentially expose users to harmful side effects.

10.4.2. DHEA

Dehydroepiandrosterone (DHEA) is a hormone that's been marketed for its anti-aging and strength-enhancing properties. But research doesn't support these claims. Moreover, its usage is banned in most competitive sports.

10.5. Summary: Supplement Smart

It's crucial to approach supplements with a degree of skepticism and informed judgement. There's no magic pill or powder to skyrocket you to your athletic goals - that territory belongs to adequate training, rest, and a balanced diet. However, when used thoughtfully and with wisdom, supplements can provide that extra push on your journey to athletic excellence.

Athletes should always remember that supplements are tools to enhance an already sound nutrition and training plan. They're not standalone solutions, and they certainly can't compensate for poor dietary habits or suboptimal training. And when in doubt, seek the advice of a dietitian or a health professional well-versed in sports nutrition.

Chapter 11. Future of Sports Nutrition: Trends and Innovations

The dynamic landscape of sports nutrition is increasingly becoming an arena of cutting-edge research and innovation, as scientists, nutritionists, and sports enthusiasts alike endeavor to unlock the ineffable secrets of the human body. Amid continuous revelations of how different foods, macronutrients, micronutrients, and their timings influence athletic performance, recovery, and overall well-being, the future of sports nutrition looks both promising and fascinating.

11.1. The Macronutrient Revolution: More Than Just Proteins

Traditionally, proteins have heralded an inordinately large share of the athlete's plate, primarily due to their well-recognized role in muscle synthesis and repair. Nevertheless, recent studies suggest that an inclusive approach, balancing all macronutrients – proteins, carbohydrates, and fats, could significantly enhance performance and recovery.

Carbohydrates are being appreciated more for their critical function of providing glucose - the primary fuel for intense exercise activities, while fats, particularly omega-3 fatty acids, are being recognized for reducing inflammation and accelerating post-workout recovery. Future innovations are likely to further investigate the ideal proportions of these macronutrients and their timings for different sports, potentially paving the way for personalized sports nutrition plans.

11.2. Rise of Microbiome Manipulation

Our gut microbiome, housing billions of microbes, is continually interacting with what we eat, influencing various physiological processes ranging from nutrient absorption to immune function. Emerging research suggests that modifying this microbiome – through foods rich in probiotics and prebiotics – could optimize these processes and potentially bolster athletic performances. Are we soon going to see bacteria-guided dietary prescriptions for athletes? Only time will tell!

11.3. Nutri-Genomics: Personalizing Sports Nutrition

As genetics increasingly becomes a determinant of sports prowess, scientists have started exploring its interplay with nutrition - a field known as nutri-genomics. Our genetic makeup can influence how our bodies metabolize different foods, which, in turn, can affect our athletic performance, recovery, and overall health. Tailoring an athlete's diet based on his/her genetic profile could unlock enormous potential benefits.

Already, organizations are offering gene-directed dietary plans, a trend set to continue in the future, with potentially increased precision and efficacy. However, this highly promising field rests on the pillars of extensive research, stringent regulation, and ethical considerations, ensuring athletes reap benefits without compromise.

11.4. Plant-Power: Veganism in Sports

Despite the longstanding belief that meat is indispensable for athletes, growing evidence suggests that plant-based diets can, in fact, support excellent athletic performance and recovery. This revelation, combined with environmental and ethical concerns, is prompting an increasing number of athletes to turn to veganism.

Plant-based diets, rich in antioxidants, can reduce inflammation and oxidative stress associated with intense physical exertion. They also offer a wide mix of carbohydrates, proteins, and healthy fats. Future research and innovation will likely focus on plant-sourced proteins and their bioavailability, besides further investigating the long-term effects of veganism in sports.

11.5. Tech-Inspired Nutritional Innovation

Just as technology is transforming sports training and performance measurement, it is also making significant strides in the realm of nutrition. Innovative tools capable of analyzing an individual's nutritional status and real-time nutrient needs can lead to more accurate diet advice and prompt course corrections. AI-driven apps providing personalized meal plans and wearable-tech monitoring hydration levels are some of the early manifestations of this integration.

Additionally, advancements in food tech might revolutionize the sports nutrition industry by creating nutrient-rich, performance-enhancing foods that are more sustainable and possibly even tailored to individual athletes.

11.6. Sustainable Sports Nutrition

With the growing realization that our food choices impact our planet's health, sustainability is evolving as a significant trend in the future of sports nutrition. Athletes, nutritional advisors, and sports bodies are increasingly advocating for diets minimizing environmental impact without compromising nutritional requirements.

This trend is likely to spur development in plant-based foods, alternative proteins (such as insects or lab-grown meat), and farming practices optimizing resource utilization.

11.7. Focus on Hydration

While nutrition strategies often revolve around food, the role of hydration is increasingly being recognized as an integral aspect of sports performance and recovery. Innovations are gravitating toward formulating beverages that optimally replenish water and electrolytes lost during workouts, tailoring to individual athletes' unique requirements.

Water isn't the only concern – novel hydration strategies are exploring natural sources of electrolytes, the use of carbohydrates to enhance absorption and fluid retention, and the precise timing of hydration for peak performance. The future hydration plans will certainly be more science-backed, personalized, and targeted.

The future of sports nutrition is complex, nuanced, and decidedly exciting with these trends and innovations shaping it. Given the rapid influx of new information, athletes and those aspiring for healthier lifestyles can anticipate nutrition regimens that are personalized, science-backed, plant-forward, and thoroughly nuanced, optimizing their health and performance. As we march ahead into this promising future, one element remains uncontested –

the enduring relevance of moderation, balance, and variety in our diets. Eating is not just for sustenance; it is a celebration of life, health, and, in the context of sports, an expression of our athletic spirit.